Phoenix Strategies

*Intelligence On How To Recover
From Past Hurts*

Sensei Paul David

Copyright Page

Phoenix Strategies: Intelligence On
How To Recover From Past Hurts,
by Sensei Paul David

Copyright © 2022

All rights reserved.

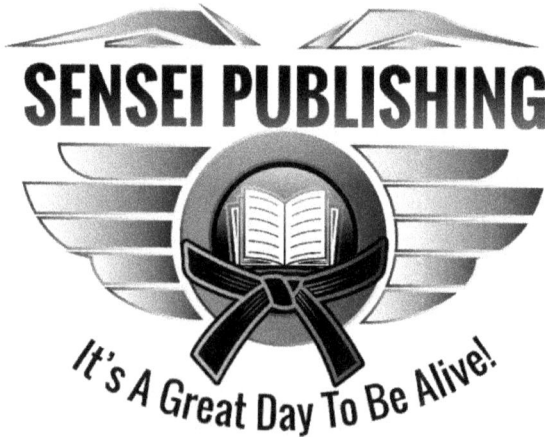

SENSEI PUBLISHING

It's A Great Day To Be Alive!

www.senseipublishing.com

@senseipublishing
senseipublishing

Get/Share Our FREE All-Ages Mental Health Book Now!

FREE Self-Development Book for Every Family

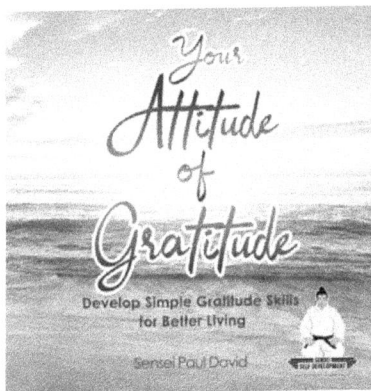

senseiselfdevelopment.senseipublishing.com

Click Below or Search Amazon for Another Book In This Series

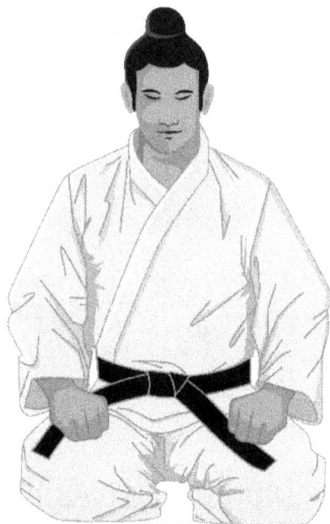

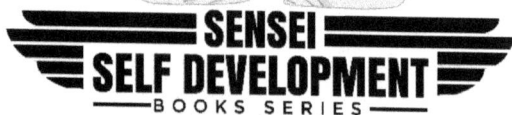

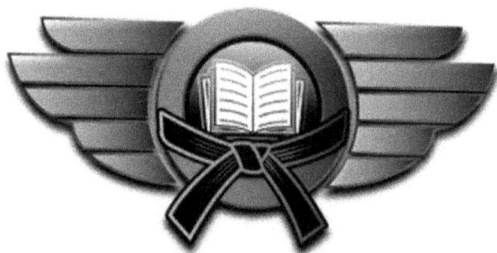

Join Our Publishing Journey!

If you would like to receive FUTURE FREE BOOKS and get to know us better, please click www.senseipublishing.com and join our newsletter by entering your email address in the pop-up box.

Follow Our Blog: senseipauldavid.ca

Follow/Like/Subscribe: Facebook, Instagram, YouTube: @senseipublishing

Scan the QR Code with your phone or tablet

to follow us on social media: Like / Subscribe / Follow

Thank You from The Author: Sensei Paul David

Before we dive in, I would like to thank you for picking up this book from among the many other similar books out there. Thank you for choosing to invest in my book. That means everything to me.

Now that you are here, I ask you to stick with me as we take your self-discovery journey together. I promise to make our time together valuable and worthwhile.

In the pages ahead, you will find some areas of information and practices more helpful than others - and that is great! I encourage you to apply what works best for you. You will benefit from the knowledge that you gain and the ensuing exciting transformation of character.

Enjoy!

Table of Contents

Foreword

A past... we all have it. Sometimes, it is full of regrets because of our mistakes. For others, it is full of torturous experiences because of the abuses they have suffered. If we are all given a chance, we would like to be given an eraser that could wipe away some parts of our past, but it is not possible.

In *Phoenix Strategies*, Paul masterfully explains the reasons it hurts so much when we think about certain events in our past. He acknowledges the pain but also provides research-based solutions to help you recover from the trauma. This is a must-read for anyone desiring to live a happy life after suffering disappointments, pain, and regret as a result of past experiences.

Introduction

"The past is behind, learn from it. The future is ahead, prepare for it. The present is here, live it."

Thomas S. Monson

Regardless of how beautiful or ugly your past is, you cannot afford to base your present or future on it. If you have a beautiful past, do not let it get into your head because it might prompt you to make mistakes that will make your future full of sadness. On the other hand, if you had a terrible past, regardless of how horrible it was, the best thing you can do for yourself is to let it go.

It is impossible to enjoy all the wonderful experiences the future offers you unless you are willing to let go of the past. This book is dedicated to everyone struggling with one hurt because of the traumatic events they have experienced. I hope you find healing through your interaction with this material.

Chapter One:
Why Does It Still Hurt?

Learn from yesterday, live for today, hope for tomorrow. The important thing is not to stop questioning."

Albert Einstein

One of the shocking things about grief is that it comes back out of nowhere sometimes, just when you thought you had overcome the hurt. The truth is that past hurts do not disappear overnight. You need to accept this reality in your journey towards healing.

Possible Reasons You Still Hurt

Some overzealous people may tell you to let go of the hurt, as though the pain does not exist. Indeed, they have good intentions but the approach is wrong. You cannot experience complete healing from a traumatic experience, immediately after it happens. However, it is a problem when the pain lingers for a long time. Below are some of the plausible reasons you still hurt several months following a traumatic event:

You Are Living In Denial

One of the reasons people struggle to recover from traumatic events is that they are living in denial. This is usually the case with divorce or a painful heartbreak. This is the first diagnostic test to consider when you find it difficult to let go of a burden from the past. It hurts, especially when you are somehow hoping that the person will realize his or her mistake and come back to you. According to statistics by DivorceMag.com, up to 50% of people who got divorced regretted their decision.

The stats may give you hope but the fact that they regretted the decision does not mean they are willing to go back to their previous partners. So, the chances are great that your ex will never return to you. One of the attributes of love is allowing people to do what is best for them. If your ex feels that there is someone else out there that will make him or her happy, you should love him or her enough to allow them to do what is best for them. For the sake of your mental health, do not expect the people who left you to come back.

You Have Not Processed The Event

Processing a traumatic event is not the easiest of tasks but you have to do it to move on. Were you sacked or did you lose a loved one? Did the love of your life walk away from you at the point you needed him or her the most? Were you raped or abused by someone so dear to you? These are a few examples of terrible situations that happen in this crazy world. No one wants to experience them but they are part and parcel of life.

If you continue to avoid processing the event because you do not want to get hurt all over again, you will make it more challenging to recover from the event. According to the author, Bessel van der Kolk, in *The Body Keeps The Score,* one of the ways you can recover from a torturous past event is by summoning the courage to process the event. It is never an easy road but it is a journey you have to embark on for long-term peace of mind. Let go of your fear and disassemble the hurt by processing it to arrive at a positive conclusion.

You Are Still Angry

Many people fail to admit that they are still angry with the people who hurt them, which enslaves them to negative emotions. We will carry out further analysis on this aspect in subsequent chapters of this book. If you keep pretending that you are not hurt or annoyed by something someone did to you, you will never experience complete and thorough healing. Every time you remember the person or event, you will feel as though a dagger is cutting through your heart.

You do not deserve that kind of emotional torture. Free yourself from it by acknowledging the hurt and taking the next step to forgiving that person. The fact that you refuse to forgive the person will not hold the individual back in most cases. It will even hurt you more when the person moves on while you are still hurting and angry. Acknowledge the hurt and move on. Admit what the person did to you or that the event caused you pain. If you continue to deny that you are annoyed, nothing will change.

You Have The Wrong People Around You

Even when you are willing to let go and move on after a disappointment, the wrong group of people around you will make it difficult to recover from the trauma. There are various ways people do this. Some people do this by taunting you and reminding you of the mistakes that led to your failure. This happens, especially when you have been arrogant or rude to such people during your heyday. Some individuals will not forgive you, thereby making life miserable for you.

On the other hand, some people will discourage you from forgiving the person that hurt you. Usually, they do this because they want to protect your interests but it is always counterproductive. No one should be allowed to keep you in bondage by fuelling the pain through their insistence on you not forgiving an offender. Let them understand that you appreciate their commitment to you but you will be happier and healthier by letting go of the hurt, which requires forgiveness.

You Have Not Found A Replacement

Moving on is seamless when you can quickly find a way of replacing what was lost with something or someone else. For example, if you lose your job amidst a controversial decision, finding another job will most likely keep you busy enough to stop you from ruminating on how you lost your previous role. In the same way, getting into another relationship is a faster healing process after a heartbreak. The love and care of the new person in your life is a perfect tonic to cure the emotional turmoil of the past relationship.

Nonetheless, you have to be careful. It is not recommended to rush into another relationship without fully processing what transpired in your previous escapade. Did you do things that frustrated your ex, and that led to irreconcilable differences? You should ask yourself such honest questions so that what happened in the previous relationship will not repeat itself. However, you should never get to a point where you feel you are not good enough for anyone. Work on yourself when necessary but no one has the right to treat you like trash.

Chapter Two:
Stop The Denial!
You Are Hurt!

"Yesterday's the past, tomorrow's the future, but today is a gift. That's why it's called the present."

Bil Keane

One of the reasons that were mentioned in the last section regarding why people still feel the pain of a past event is denial. It comes in various forms. Regardless of what form it takes, it will hamper you from making the best of your life. In this chapter, we will discuss the various forms of denials that make it difficult for people to let go of past hurt.

Forms Of Denial

Some of the forms of denial that exist among people battling with demons from their past are:

Refusal To Admit Vulnerability

Based on a 2018 study published in *Frontiers in Psychology*, three of the common signs of a person engaging in self-criticism are:

- Not wanting to show weakness
- Feeling guilty or angry
- Feeling like a burden

When people are holding on to their past, they might not want to admit the fact that they are hurt because they do not want their friends and family to know that they still carry the burden of the torturous event. When the people around them counsel them to forgive a person that broke their heart, they will deny it. They will claim that they have moved on only to shed hot tears when they are alone.

If this is your story, it is high time you stop the deceit. It is not advisable to allow the fake display of strength by many people in the world to affect you. Many people that act as though they are strong and impeccable are broken on the inside. When you fail to admit your vulnerability, you are only pretending to be another superman. Guess what? Superman only exists in the world of comics. Well, even in that world, Superman is vulnerable to kryptonite!

Of course, you cannot share what you are going through with everybody. Yet, it is okay to cry in front of the people that matter. You are a human being. So, being vulnerable and weak sometimes does not make you useless. It is the admittance of vulnerability that will make you meet the people that can help you heal completely. No one will know you are drowning if you fail to cry out for help. Displaying your vulnerability is also one of the most effective ways to become a leader. Your experience convinces others that you have been in their shoes and have what it takes to help and lead them.

Denial Of The Need For Support And Encouragement

You are only deceiving yourself if you claim that you do not need to be encouraged sometimes. Indeed, self-motivation is best because you can always count on it. You are the source of encouragement to yourself when you practice self-motivation. Therefore, you can always inspire and encourage yourself. Some of the greatest achievers in the world today are self-motivators. They have been down several times but they never gave up. Some world-renowned entrepreneurs have failed in the past but they did not allow the disappointments to define them or determine their future.

Nonetheless, when you read their stories, you will notice that they also had people who encouraged and supported them during their low moments. This is the benefit of having positive and encouraging people around you. You might not realize the importance of such people when things are going well for you but you will be glad you have them when you are struggling and disappointed. However, some people never get the help and support they need because they keep denying that they need help. Such people drown without a trace but they could have been saved if only they had asked.

In a world where consent is becoming increasingly important, people will be wary of helping you if you do not ask them to because no one wants to waste effort. No one wants to try to help, only to be insulted or embarrassed. So, you must be humble enough to seek help when you know that you need it. Of course, good friends will try to help you even when you have not asked them, especially when you have shown support for them during their stormy days. Yet, they might not know what you need unless you ask.

Refusal To Surrender

There is no doubt that resilience is a great virtue. Nonetheless, it is wise to know when to surrender. In the words of Lalah Delia:

"If you walk away from a toxic, negative, abusive, one-sided, dead-end low vibrational relationship or friendship – you won."

Sometimes, you will be proud of yourself for not giving up, but other times staying longer and holding on will lead to regret. You need people to succeed and live the happy life they desire but your success and happiness should never hinge on anyone. That is too much power to give to one human being. When people are in love, they claim that their spouse is their source of joy. Indeed, your spouse should make you happy but he or she should never be your *source* of joy.

If the person should choose to walk away from your life, you might be too devastated to recover. People always promise themselves forever, but some "forevers" only last for two years. So, even when you are in a relationship with someone you love, it is not recommended that you make the person your everything, because people change and crazy things happen.

Enough Is Enough

You cannot go on like this. You just have to tell yourself that you deserve to be happy. It is time to let go of the burden of the past by ending your overdue stay in the prison of denial. You have nothing to gain from pretending to be impeccable. Every human being has its weaknesses. It is time to admit that you were hurt by the action of your former boss, ex, parents, family member, or friends.

Your healing begins from that point on. You are the hero of the story of your life. It is time to stop blaming yourself or hoping that the people that left your life will come back. Denial has not been working, so, why not try something different? Why not acknowledge the pain and hurt to move to the next level in life?

Chapter Three: Leveraging The Power Of Forgiveness

"The future depends on what we do in the present."

Mahatma Gandhi

Starting that beautiful future you crave begins by letting go of the hurt of the past. You might have made mistakes that messed up your life but you have to forgive yourself. This rule also applies to the people who hurt you. In this chapter, we will discuss the health benefits of forgiveness and how it can help you to lift the burdens of the past that weigh you down.

Forgive For Your Own Sake

If there is one thing I have helped many people achieve in their lives, it is forgiving others. In some cases, the offense was grievous and painful. Yet, I know that the person that forgives others is the true beneficiary of the act. I have understood from a tender age that forgiveness is non-negotiable for anyone who wants to be happy, and that is why it is my only option, regardless of how bad I may feel because of something someone had done to me. Besides, studies have shown that forgiveness is beneficial to our mental health.

For example, based on a study by the John Hopkins Hospital, forgiveness offers several health benefits. In my college days, I had a friend who was raped as a teenager, by a trusted friend. Expectedly, her heart was broken. Unfortunately, the intercourse led to pregnancy. She was not ready to be a mother and she could not imagine getting married to the guy. So, she aborted the baby. What she went through embittered her. She wished the guy would experience unfortunate events that would make him experience the pain he had caused her. However, she did not see any evil affecting him, and this frustrated her more.

If you are one of those people who believes in Karma, it is recommended that you reconsider your position. The truth about life is that calamity befalls both good and bad people. So, it is not tenable to claim that a person experiencing turbulent periods is paying for his or her sins. It is not healthy to expect the downfall of people that hurt you because it might not happen, which will destabilize and hurt you even more. Therefore, what is best for you is to forgive people regardless of what they do to you.

Forgiveness is the Only Option

The aforementioned lady eventually chose to forgive the guy. She stopped wishing him evil and this improved her mental health. She was happier and was able to focus on making the best of her life. Her experience is in line with a 2020 study that showed that forgiveness leads to the elimination of resentment and anger. In a world that is full of disappointments, you must avoid anger and resentment because they can be weaponized to make your life miserable.

When you are resentful and angry, the chances are good that you will seek vengeance, which can backfire. Some people in jail today find themselves there because they refused to forgive someone that hurt them. They took their pound of flesh and got into trouble with the law enforcement agency. No one can ruin your life unless you allow them to. The fact that someone hurt you and denied you opportunities does not mean that you cannot still succeed.

When you choose to forgive, the chances of doing something rash are eliminated. It will also help you to focus on your growth, which enhances your chance of success. Therefore, forgiveness is for your own good. This reality is the reason you should see forgiveness as your only option when people hurt you. Practice it often and you can be sure that you will see a tremendous difference in the quality of your life.

No One Deserves To Be Forgiven

I once saw a misleading quote that stated that forgiveness is only for people who deserve it. Many undiscerning people subscribe to this quote but it is misleading. Who deserves to be forgiven? Is there forgiveness unless there is an offense? My point is that we all hurt people sometimes, even without meaning to. So, there is no such thing as forgiving the people that deserve it. If you fail to forgive others, it will make a monster out of you.

Bitterness will only drag you down and make you a harbinger of negative emotions. It is not healthy to categorize offenses into pardonable and unpardonable. Remember that forgiveness is for your own good. Based on a 2010 study, forgiveness improves our mental health. So, quit thinking that you will only forgive the people that deserve it because no one deserves to be forgiven.

You will be hurt when people offend you and I am not denying that. One of the reasons it hurts a lot is when you are not expecting the person to hurt you. Betrayals hurt more because it comes from people you trusted. Yet, it is in your best interest to forgive people, regardless of what they have done to you. In the words of Lewis Smedes:

"To forgive is to set a prisoner free and to discover that the prisoner was you."

Actively Seek Reconciliation

Many people make the mistake of waiting for the person that hurt them to seek their forgiveness before they forgive them. If you understand the importance of forgiving others, you will never wait for them to seek your forgiveness, before you forgive them. According to Jonathan Huie,

"Forgive others not because they deserve forgiveness, but because you deserve peace."

Do you want peace of mind? Actively seek reconciliation. You might be wondering why I am talking about reconciliation when we have been discussing forgiveness throughout this section. Unknown to many people, reconciliation is the greatest proof of forgiveness. Note that reconciliation does not mean that you have to continue the relationship, especially when the other party does not want it.

It implies that you will never wish the person evil and will help the person if the opportunity arises. It will also mean that you are willing to have meaningful conversations with the person if there is a reason for it. One of the signs of maturity is the ability to create a platform for forgiveness. Make it your goal to seek reconciliation. You will be happier about it.

Chapter Four:
Stay Away

"You cannot expect to live a positive life if you hang around negative people."

Joel Osteen

Reconciling with people is vital. However, sometimes, you might have to stay away from some people, at least for some time, to be in good shape before you can see them again. This approach can save you from many stressful circumstances. In this chapter, we will discuss the importance of staying away from people that can make it difficult for you to let go of your past.

Never Overestimate Yourself

Some years ago, I was in love with a lady. She was my world. I could not imagine a future without her and I made sure to remind her as much as I could. However, for reasons I still cannot explain even till now, she told me she did not want to be with me anymore. I was devastated. My world was crashing around me and I did not know what to do. Out of desperation, I began to buy her gifts to convince her that I truly loved her and would do anything to make her happy.

She kept accepting the gifts but would turn me down anytime I asked her to reconsider the decision. This went on for some months until I finally told myself the truth – she'd moved on. That relationship was now a part of my past. It was a bitter pill to swallow but I realized that I was hurting myself more by begging her to return. Each rejection hurt more than the previous one. I was frustrated and could hardly concentrate on anything without remembering how much I wanted her to be my wife.

Initially, I thought I could handle being around her despite her rejection. However, it was just not working. I was hurt even more and thoughts of assaulting her ran through my mind sometimes. At that point, I realized I needed to stay away from her. That was the only way I could find the space to heal and forgive her. Staying around her only reminded me of how much I loved her and the pain of her failure to reciprocate my love was unbearable. Overestimating my ability to handle the heartbreak would have been a mistake I would regret years down the line.

Have Your Space

You must recognize when to step back. One of the reasons some people struggle to let go of the past is that they are still close to the people that hurt them when they have yet to heal from the pain. Isolation is needed once in a while to have that breathing space to rethink and reflect on certain areas of your life. If you refuse to stay away from some people, it can damage your self-esteem and ruin other aspects of your life.

The period of staying away also helps you to reduce the tension around the issue. You will not see the person, as such cutting out the chance of hearing something that will make you angry and frustrated all over again. No one should have the ability to make you angry or frustrated at will.

Be astute enough to know when leaving is the solution. Your mental health is at stake. You will only regret it if you waste time waiting for someone to love and accept you. If the person ends up turning you down, you will rue the time wasted.

Time is a precious commodity you should never waste on anyone or anything that makes you feel worthless.

Heal From Afar

The healing period after a disappointment or heartbreak is not for staying alone and reflecting on what happened, while alone. If care is not taken, you might start thinking negative thoughts that will lead to depression. Therefore, it is recommended that you spend that period reading books and listening to empowering podcasts that will strengthen your resolve to move on and try something new.

No matter how devastating a setback is, you can recover from it and make the best of the remaining part of your life. Nonetheless, you might struggle with this reality when you are hurting. The pain and disappointment of that moment might make it challenging for you to find reasons to imagine a better future. Still, the reality is that there is so much in store for you if you do not give up.

These are the kind of empowering thoughts you will have when you read books and podcasts. You can ask your friends and family to recommend useful ones to you. Reading and listening to podcasts are two vital sources of learning and inspiration for me. While staying away from the people that hurt you, fill your mind with empowering and inspiring thoughts that will help you recover your smile.

No One Is Irreplaceable

The loss of a loved one is one of the most challenging and traumatic events that make many people miserable. According to a 2016 study, the loss of a loved one is one of the major reasons people indulge in self-neglect. Despite the pain of losing a loved one, the fact is that no one is irreplaceable. You might not find a person with the same qualities and personality but you can always find someone who will carry out the role you desire from a person.

Let me explain this in football terms. Ronaldinho Gaucho is one of the most skillful players the world of football has ever seen. During his prime years at Barcelona, he was almost unstoppable unless you kicked him. The club won trophies as a result of his brilliance and he rightly won the award of the best footballer of the year. However, Barcelona soon appointed a new coach who decided to sell him to another club. It was a shock to many football fans because they felt Ronaldinho was irreplaceable.

Guess what? After he left, the burgeoning Lionel Messi became a beast. He humiliated opponents and took the club to greater heights. Ronaldinho and Messi do not have the same skill set. One is right-footed while the other is left-footed. However, Messi arguably offered more to the Club than Ronaldinho ever did. Never let anyone think they are irreplaceable in your life. If they choose to replace you, replace them too. You deserve to be treated with love and valued. Do not settle for less.

Chapter Five: Mindfulness To The Rescue

"We are all here for some reason. Stop being a prisoner of your past. Become the architect of your future."

Robin Sharma

In recent times, the West has been incorporating some Eastern practices to improve the quality of life of people. One of these practices is mindfulness. Note that mindfulness is not the same as meditation even though they share certain similarities. In this chapter, we will explore how you can leverage mindfulness to keep the demons from your past at bay.

Here And Now

It is always frustrating to see people whose attention is divided when you are speaking with them. In this digital age where people spend a considerable time of the day on their phones, concentrating has never been more challenging. Many parents work on their phones at home, reducing the quality of time they spend with their kids. This presents the wrong image to some children who begin to think that their friends and other people care about them more than their parents, simply because of the quality of attention they get elsewhere.

This lack of attention can also ruin a marriage. You do not want to speak to your partner when he or she is surfing the Internet, especially when you want to discuss something serious with him or her. It has gotten so bad for some people that they are addicted to social media. It is almost as though the world has ended if they have not visited Twitter, Instagram, or Facebook in a day. This has also led to the discovery of a psychological dysfunction known as the Fear Of Missing Out (FOMO). People battling this condition are anxious because they feel that they are missing out on a novel experience online.

Meanwhile, the absence of mindfulness is hurting us in terms of productivity and well-being. According to a 2013 study that examined the effect of mindfulness on psychological health, mindfulness enhances subjective well-being and behavioral regulation. It also reduces emotional reactivity. Therefore, it makes perfect sense to incorporate this practice into our day-to-day activities. It can make a tremendous difference even if you are not trying to wrest your life back from the demons of your past. It also promises to restore your sanity and peace of mind when you are trying to recover your smile again.

Away With The Monkey Mind

The earlier you realize the tremendous power that lies in utilizing your mind, the better for you. In the words of rapper NF:

"The mind is a powerful place, what you put in it can affect you in a powerful way."

If the human mind were a person, it would be classified as a chronic workaholic. It never stops working! Even when you are sleeping, your mind is still working and that is what translates into dreams and nightmares. Your mind is a wild animal that does not want to be tamed so that it can keep jumping wherever it wants. This is what the Buddha called the "Monkey Mind." It is that state of restlessness where your mind jumps from one thought to another.

Meanwhile, this autopilot mode is not healthy for you because it can make you focus on negative thoughts that can ruin your mood. So, you need to wrest control back from your mind, and mindfulness is crucial in this regard. Mindfulness is all about ensuring that you are focused on what you are doing currently. For example, when you practice mindfulness, you will enjoy your meal by focusing solely on it, rather than eating while thinking about your presentation in your office, which can lead to anxiety.

Defeating The Demons Of The Past

Banishing images and memories of the past from your mind is impossible because of the active nature of the mind. However, you can reconstruct the events with mindfulness. The following tips will help you in this regard:

Be Deliberate

The key aspect when it comes to mindfulness is being deliberate. This is what will make you discover your recurrent negative thoughts about the past. Based on a 2016 study that examined the impact of mindfulness-based therapy on depression, the result showed that it helps curb recurrent depressive thoughts.

Begin by discovering those recurrent thoughts that make you angry, frustrated, or depressed. This is the beginning of your healing process. The moment you can identify those thoughts, you are not far from turning a corner. The hidden enemy is the most dangerous. So, once you discover the recurrent thoughts that ruin your mood, you are beginning to disarm those demons tormenting you from your past.

Ask Questions

After discovering your recurrent negative thoughts, it is recommended that you ask yourself critical questions that will give you a different perspective. For example, you can ask yourself what you would have done if it were your friend that was holding onto the past. Would you tell him to keep sulking and crying or would you tell him to move on? If your answer is the latter, doctor, heal yourself! Take your prescription!

With the aid of mental imagery, get out of yourself and take a good look at your sorry and sulking self. Tell yourself what you would have told a sulking self. You will find yourself seeing things from a different perspective as you do this. This is the power of mindfulness.

Remember Your Goals

The past has a way of making us forget about the future we promised ourselves. Did you not say you were going to change the world with your business? What about your plans to take many people out of poverty? Will you be able to achieve these goals when you are struggling to concentrate because of the things that happened in your past?

Is that man or woman worth sacrificing your future for? Of course not! No disappointment should ever make you feel as though your life has come to an end. As you meditate, focus on your goals and remember the reasons you were inspired to achieve them in the first place. According to a study involving 2,000 participants, achievement goals are effective for defeating negative thoughts. Keep your eye on the ball!

Change The Narrative

You will begin to feel empowered as you start reminding yourself of the goals you plan to achieve. As you picture how you will feel when you finally achieve them, your heart will start racing. Take a deep breath to let it all sink in. Dust yourself off and roll up your sleeves. It is time for work! Were you sacked? Apply for a job or start your own business! Did you experience a divorce? Tell yourself that you deserve to be happy with or without a partner. Change the narrative! Get to work!

Chapter Six: Creating Positive Energy Through Gratitude

"Yesterday is gone. Tomorrow is yet to come. We only have today. Let us begin."

Mother Teresa

The topsy-turvy nature of life makes it easy to switch from a positive mood to a negative one within an hour. This possibility is one of the reasons the pursuit of happiness is elusive for many people. In this chapter, we will discuss how you can take advantage of gratitude to banish the demons from your past and live a happy life.

www.ingramcontent.com/pod-product-compliance
Lightning Source LLC
Chambersburg PA
CBHW071240020426
42333CB00015B/1562